GOUT DIET COOKBOOK

Delicious Recipes For Managing Uric Acid, Reducing Inflammation, And Alleviating Pain

DR ELIAN GRIFFIN

Copyright © [Elian Griffin] [2024]. All rights reserved.

Without the publisher's prior written consent, no portion of this publication may be copied, distributed, or transmitted in any way, including by photocopying, recording, or other mechanical or electronic means, with the exception of brief quotations used in all critical reviews.

DISCLAIMER

The nutritional recommendations and recipes in this book are meant solely for informative reasons. They are not meant to replace the counsel, diagnosis, or care of a qualified medical expert. If you have any doubts about a medical condition or dietary requirements, you should always see your physician or another trained healthcare expert.

All reasonable efforts have been taken by the author and publisher to ensure that the information contained in this book is correct as of the date of publication. Recommendations may alter, though, as medical knowledge is always changing. When using any of the recipes or instructions found here, the user assumes all liability and assumes no risk, whether personal or otherwise. People who have certain dietary requirements or medical issues should speak with a healthcare provider for personalized guidance. The given recipes are only ideas; you may need to adjust them to suit your own nutritional needs, tastes, and tolerances.

When you use this book, you agree to release the publisher, the author, and their representatives from any liability for any claims, damages, liabilities, costs, or expenditures resulting from your use of the book.

TABLE OF CONTENTS

ABOUT THE BOOK

The "Gout Diet Cookbook" is an invaluable tool created to provide people with gout with thorough dietary strategies and doable meal plans. Gout is a type of arthritis that is brought on by the buildup of uric acid crystals in joints, and if left untreated, can have a severe negative influence on quality of life. A carefully planned diet is essential to managing gout, and this cookbook acts as a roadmap for navigating the complexities of eating gout-friendly.

This book starts with a detailed introduction to gout, explaining its causes and emphasizing the critical role of nutrition in reducing symptoms and preventing recurrences. By emphasizing the fundamentals of the gout diet, including foods to avoid and those beneficial for managing the condition, the cookbook offers clear guidelines for creating meals that support overall health. Understanding the importance of diet in managing gout is imperative, as dietary choices directly influence uric acid levels and subsequent flare-ups.

This cookbook is unique in that it takes a pragmatic approach to application, providing readers with the knowledge and tools they need to make the most of it. From understanding uric acid levels and creating customized dietary goals to weekly meal planning advice and necessary shopping lists, each feature is intended to make it easier for gout-aware eating to become a regular part of everyday life.

The cookbook's main attraction is its carefully planned recipes for every meal and occasion. Low-purine breakfast options, nutrient-rich salads, lean protein options, and hearty soups can all be found in the chapters devoted to breakfast, lunch, and dinner. Snack and appetizer ideas are tailored to different palates and environments so that people can always have something tasty and gout-safe to eat. Drinks and hydration tactics are also covered, including recipes for herbal infusions, and smoothies, and crucial information on alcohol intake.

Apart from recipes, the cookbook covers events and handling flare-ups. It offers direction on diet modifications during flare-ups, stressing hydration, and recuperation strategies. Lifestyle advice includes workout suggestions, stress reduction methods, and the significance of sufficient sleep and supplements for gout prevention. Frequently asked questions and common issues are also covered in detail, providing useful information on interacting with others and choosing foods.

All things considered, the "Gout Diet Cookbook" is a thorough guide for anyone attempting to manage their gout. It does this by combining informative text with useful recipes and lifestyle advice, enabling readers to take charge of their health by making educated food choices and making holistic lifestyle changes.

CHAPTER ONE

GOUT DIET INTRODUCTION

GOUT OVERVIEW

Uric acid forms when the body breaks down purines, which are substances found in foods and beverages. When uric acid levels become too high, crystals can form and deposit in the joints, causing excruciating pain, swelling, and inflammation. Gout is a type of arthritis that typically affects the big toe joints but can also occur in other joints like the ankles, knees, wrists, and elbows. Those who have gout often wake up from sleep in excruciating pain.

Gout management is a multimodal approach that includes medications to lower uric acid levels and lifestyle changes like adopting a gout-friendly diet. People can help prevent gout attacks and improve their overall quality of life by reducing purine intake and maintaining a healthy weight. Gout is a condition that can be influenced by genetics as well as lifestyle factors like diet, alcohol consumption, obesity, and certain medical conditions.

Gaining a thorough understanding of gout enables people to make educated decisions about their health. Early symptom recognition and knowledge of the influence of diet and lifestyle enable people to take proactive measures to effectively manage their condition, which includes not only listening to their doctors' advice but also implementing dietary modifications that support gout management and lower the likelihood of recurrent attacks.

DIET IS IMPORTANT IN THE MANAGEMENT OF GOUT

Purine-rich foods, such as red meat, organ meats, and some seafood, like anchovies and sardines, can raise uric acid levels and exacerbate gout attacks; on the other hand, foods low in purines, like fruits, vegetables, whole grains, and low-fat dairy products, can help lower uric acid levels and reduce the frequency of gout flare-ups. Diet is important in managing gout because certain foods can either trigger or alleviate symptoms.

Eating a balanced diet is important for overall health and can have a big impact on managing gout. People can support their body's natural ability to manage uric acid levels by concentrating on foods that are high in nutrients and low in purines. This dietary strategy can help prevent gout attacks and also help people manage their weight, which is important because obesity is a risk factor for gout.

Beyond simply avoiding purine-rich foods, a gout-friendly diet also entails drinking plenty of water, reducing alcohol, and consuming sugar-filled drinks and fructose-containing foods in moderation. Gout sufferers can improve the efficacy of their medical treatment and eventually lessen the intensity and frequency of their gout attacks by implementing these dietary changes.

FUNDAMENTALS OF A GOUT DIET

A key component of the gout diet is limiting purine-rich foods and increasing foods that help lower uric acid levels. Lean proteins, like tofu and poultry, are lower in purines than red meat and organ meats.

You should also eat a lot of fruits and vegetables, which are high in antioxidants and low in purines, as these can help reduce inflammation and support overall joint health.

Hydration is key, as water helps flush out excess uric acid from the body, reducing the risk of crystal formation in the joints.

Whole grains, like brown rice and whole wheat bread, are preferred over refined grains because they provide more fiber and essential nutrients. Low-fat dairy products, like yogurt and skim milk, are also recommended because they can help decrease uric acid levels.

The gout diet requires an understanding of portion sizes and meal planning. People can maintain stable blood sugar levels and prevent overeating, which can result in weight gain and elevated uric acid levels, by controlling portion sizes and spacing out meals throughout the day. Keeping a food journal and consulting with a registered dietitian can also help people identify trigger foods and create customized meal plans that support managing their gout.

HOW THIS COOKBOOK IS USEFUL

With its assortment of delectable recipes that are high in nutrients and low in purines, this Gout Diet Cookbook aims to make it easier for people with gout to follow a gout-friendly diet without compromising taste or enjoyment.

Each recipe is thoughtfully crafted to include ingredients that support joint health and reduce inflammation, guaranteeing that people with gout can enjoy satisfying meals while managing their condition effectively.

Using this cookbook, people can take charge of their gout management journey and improve their overall quality of life through wholesome and delectable eating habits. In addition to recipes, it provides helpful advice on grocery shopping, meal planning, and cooking techniques that maximize flavor and nutrition. It also includes information on ingredient substitutions and portion control, empowering people to make informed decisions about their diet and lifestyle.

Whether you're new to managing gout or looking for new ideas for your meal plan, this cookbook offers a wealth of useful information and delicious recipes to support your journey toward better health. It is an invaluable tool for anyone looking to broaden their culinary repertoire while following the guidelines of the gout diet. It also fosters creativity in the kitchen and offers inspiration for meals that are both health-conscious and satisfying.

HOW TO USE THIS BOOK EFFECTIVELY

Take advantage of the recipe index to browse a variety of dishes categorized by meal type, making it easier to find options that suit your preferences and dietary needs. To get the most out of this Gout Diet Cookbook, approach it strategically. Begin by becoming acquainted with the introductory sections, which lay out the fundamentals of the gout diet and offer advice for efficient meal planning.

Consider experimenting with different flavors and cuisines to keep your meals interesting and enjoyable while supporting your overall health. When choosing recipes, pay attention to ingredient lists and nutritional information to ensure they align with your gout management goals. Focus on incorporating foods that are rich in vitamins, minerals, and antioxidants and low in purines.

Organize your weekly menus and make shopping lists using the meal planning templates included in the cookbook. This will save you time and ensure that you have the ingredients you need on hand to meet your dietary goals. Don't forget to practice moderation and portion control to maintain a balanced diet that effectively supports gout management.

Through active use of the recipes and resources in this cookbook, you can change the way you eat while managing gout.

Seize the chance to try new foods and flavors that improve your overall health. Every meal you make with recipes from this cookbook is a proactive step toward better health and a higher quality of life—one delectable dish at a time.

CHAPTER TWO

ESSENTIALS OF A GOUT DIET

AN OVERVIEW OF THE CAUSES OF GOUT

Uric acid is produced when the body breaks down purines, which are found naturally in the body and some foods. When the kidneys are unable to effectively eliminate uric acid, it builds up and forms sharp, needle-like crystals in joints or surrounding tissue, causing inflammation and intense pain. Some factors that can increase the risk of developing gout include genetics, obesity, certain medical conditions, and lifestyle choices. Gout is a type of arthritis that is characterized by sudden, severe attacks of pain, redness, and tenderness in joints, frequently affecting the big toe.

To effectively manage gout, it is important to recognize its causes. Foods high in purines, such as red meat, organ meats, and some seafood, can raise uric acid levels significantly. Other factors that contribute to elevated uric acid production include alcohol, especially beer and spirits, and sugary beverages. Chronic health conditions, such as metabolic syndrome, diabetes, and hypertension, are also associated with higher uric acid levels, which can exacerbate gout symptoms. Diabetic medications, which are used to treat hypertension, can interfere with the removal of uric acid, which can lead to its buildup. Sedentary lifestyle choices, poor diets, and dehydration can further increase the risk, emphasizing the significance of comprehensive management strategies.

Gout can be prevented by dietary modifications, lifestyle changes, and medication when needed. Reducing uric acid production with medications such as febuxostat or allopurinol, as well as managing pain during attacks with anti-inflammatory drugs, can help lower uric acid levels and prevent flare-ups. Long-term management of gout requires regular monitoring of uric acid levels and adherence to treatment plans. Knowledge of the interactions between genetics, diet, and lifestyle can help people take proactive measures to prevent and effectively manage gout.

Effective gout management involves careful attention to diet, especially avoiding foods high in purines, which can raise uric acid levels. Red meats, such as beef, lamb, and pork, and organ meats, such as liver and kidneys, are high in purines and should be reduced or avoided. High-purine seafood, such as shellfish, anchovies, sardines, mackerel, and tuna, can also cause gout attacks. Processed meats and high-fructose foods, such as sugary drinks and desserts, can raise uric acid production and should be avoided to prevent flare-ups.

Wine may be a safer option in moderation, but it's important to consult a healthcare provider for personalized advice based on individual health conditions and risk factors. Reducing or eliminating alcohol intake can significantly improve overall health and manage gout. Alcohol consumption, particularly beer and spirits, is a significant contributor to gout symptoms and should be limited or avoided. Alcohol not only increases uric acid production but also impairs the kidneys' ability to excrete it, leading to its accumulation in the bloodstream.

Healthy fats such as those found in nuts and seeds, lean proteins, and low-fat or fat-free dairy products can help control weight and lessen the frequency of gout attacks. Purine-rich foods should be avoided by those with gout to better manage their symptoms and quality of life. High-fat foods, such as fried foods and full-fat dairy products, can exacerbate gout symptoms by promoting weight gain and increasing inflammation. Obesity is a known risk factor for gout, as excess body weight can lead to higher uric acid levels and decreased kidney function.

PRODUCTS TO PUT IN YOUR GOUT-FRIENDLY DIET

Low-purine foods help lower uric acid levels in the body, which helps manage and prevent flare-ups. Fruits, especially vitamin C-rich ones like cherries, oranges, and strawberries, are good because they can lower uric acid levels and reduce inflammation. Broccoli, spinach, kale, and other leafy greens are good choices because they provide important nutrients and antioxidants without adding to the body's uric acid buildup. Whole grains, like oats, brown rice, and whole wheat bread, are high in fiber and help maintain a healthy weight, which further reduces the risk of gout attacks.

Nuts and seeds, like almonds, walnuts, and flaxseeds, offer healthy fats and protein, contributing to a balanced diet and effectively managing gout symptoms. Low-fat and non-dairy alternatives, like skim milk, low-fat yogurt, and cheese, are excellent sources of protein and calcium without the high purine content found in full-fat dairy products.

Plant-based proteins, like tofu, legumes, and lentils, are excellent alternatives to animal proteins, providing necessary nutrients while minimizing the production of uric acid.

A gout-friendly diet must include adequate hydration. Drinking lots of water aids in the kidneys' removal of excess uric acid, which prevents it from crystallizing in the joints.

Herbal teas, like nettle or ginger tea, can also be included because they may have anti-inflammatory qualities. Sugar-filled drinks should be avoided in favor of water or natural fruit juices. Gout sufferers can live better lives and experience fewer and milder attacks when they follow a well-balanced diet high in low-purine foods and sufficient hydration.

THE VALUE OF HYDRATION

Maintaining adequate hydration is crucial for managing gout because it helps dilute and eliminate excess uric acid from the bloodstream, which prevents it from crystallizing in the joints. A minimum of 8 to 10 glasses of water per day can support kidney function and improve the body's excretion of uric acid, which lowers the risk of flare-ups.

Additionally, staying hydrated improves joint health overall by reducing inflammation and promoting better mobility in the joints. Water-rich foods such as celery, cucumbers, and watermelon can also help you stay hydrated throughout the day.

Unsweetened herbal teas and natural fruit juices can also help with hydration and gout management. Herbal teas, like nettle or ginger, have anti-inflammatory properties that may help with gout symptoms. Tart cherry juice, in particular, has been shown to lower uric acid levels and reduce inflammation, so it's a great addition to a gout-friendly diet. Sugary drinks, like soda, and some fruit juices, can worsen gout symptoms, so it's important to stick to hydrating, natural beverages instead of sugar-filled drinks.

Gout sufferers should prioritize their overall health, lessen the frequency of their attacks, and enhance their joint function and comfort by making drinking water a regular part of their daily routine.

It is important to monitor and maintain fluid levels, particularly during hot weather or physical activity, which can increase fluid loss and the risk of dehydration. Signs of dehydration, such as fatigue, dark urine, and dry mouth, should be addressed promptly by increasing water intake.

Carrying a water bottle and setting reminders to drink water throughout the day can help ensure consistent hydration.

EXAMPLE OF A BEGINNER'S MEAL PLAN

A well-balanced diet for gout management should include foods high in nutrients and low in purines, as well as plenty of water. For breakfast, try a bowl of oatmeal with a few almonds and fresh berries, served with a glass of skim milk or a dairy substitute. This meal supplies fiber, vitamins, and protein without raising blood uric acid levels. Alternatively, you could have a smoothie with low-fat yogurt, spinach, bananas, and a little tart cherry juice for a wholesome and energizing breakfast.

A light but satisfying lunch option is a salad dressed with olive oil and lemon juice that includes grilled chicken breast, cherry tomatoes, cucumbers, and mixed greens; serving it with quinoa or brown rice on the side adds extra fiber and energy. Another option is a stir-fried vegetable dish that includes tofu, bell peppers, broccoli, and carrots; all served over brown rice or whole-grain noodles. These meals are high in vitamins, minerals, and antioxidants that help manage symptoms of gout and support general health.

Starters can effectively manage their symptoms of gout by following this meal plan, which includes a variety of delicious and nutritious foods. For dinner, baked salmon with a side of steamed asparagus and sweet potatoes can provide a balanced meal rich in omega-3 fatty acids, vitamins, and fiber. Alternatively, a lentil and vegetable stew served with whole-grain bread offers a hearty and nourishing option. Adding a side salad or roasted vegetables can enhance the meal's nutritional profile. Throughout the day, make sure to drink plenty of water and think about having a glass of tart cherry juice.

CHAPTER THREE

MEAL PLANNING

CREATING OBJECTIVES FOR GOUT TREATMENT

Setting attainable goals is the first step towards effective gout management. Write down your main goals, such as minimizing the frequency and intensity of gout attacks, keeping a healthy weight, and enhancing general joint health. Then, break these bigger goals down into smaller, more doable tasks, like drinking a certain amount of water a day or increasing your intake of low-purine foods. Track your progress regularly and make necessary adjustments to your goals to stay motivated and focused on your long-term health.

Aim for at least 30 minutes of moderate activity most days of the week. Including lifestyle changes is essential for managing gout. Pay particular attention to dietary changes, such as cutting back on high-purine foods like red meat and shellfish and increasing consumption of fruits, vegetables, and whole grains.

Additionally, make a regular physical activity commitment to support weight management and overall wellness. Exercise can help lower uric acid levels and reduce the risk of gout attacks.

The secret to managing your gout is to be consistent and to keep an eye out for potential triggers or patterns in your food and symptom diary. This will help you make informed decisions about your diet and lifestyle. Frequent check-ups with your healthcare provider will also guarantee that your uric acid levels are within the target range and that your treatment plan is still working.

KNOWING THE LEVELS OF URIC ACID

Maintaining a healthy lifestyle and minimizing the risk of gout flare-ups requires an understanding of uric acid levels, which are a byproduct of purine metabolism. High blood uric acid levels can cause crystals to form in the joints, resulting in excruciating gout attacks. Regular blood tests can help monitor your uric acid levels, providing important information to guide your dietary and lifestyle choices.

The management of uric acid levels is largely dependent on diet. Eating foods low in purines, like fruits, vegetables, and whole grains, can help lower the production of uric acid. Drinking plenty of water can also help the kidneys excrete uric acid. Reducing alcohol intake, especially beer, and avoiding sugary drinks can also help maintain healthy uric acid levels.

It's important to follow your healthcare provider's recommendations and take medications as prescribed to maintain optimal uric acid levels and prevent gout attacks. Some people may require medication to manage their uric acid levels effectively.

WEEKLY GUIDE TO MEAL PLANNING

Meal planning is an essential part of managing gout. To begin, make a weekly menu consisting of a range of low-purine foods, such as fruits, vegetables, lean proteins, and whole grains.

To ensure nutritional adequacy, plan your meals to include balanced portions of protein, carbohydrates, and healthy fats. You can find delicious and simple-to-make gout-friendly recipes by searching online or in cookbooks.

Successful meal planning requires organization. Set aside time each week to plan your meals and make a thorough shopping list based on your menu. To save time during hectic workdays, think about prepping some ingredients, like chopping vegetables or cooking grains. Batch cooking and freezing portions can also be useful for easy and quick meals throughout the week.

A healthy weight is important for managing gout, so be mindful of portion sizes and avoid overeating. Every so often, review and tweak your meal plans based on your progress and any changes in your condition. Adding flexibility and variety to your meal planning will help you stay motivated and avoid boredom while adhering to your gout-friendly diet.

ESSENTIALS FOR A SHOPPING LIST

Making a thorough shopping list is crucial to following a gout-friendly diet. Begin by enumerating every item required for your weekly meal plan, emphasizing foods low in purines, such as lean proteins like fish and chicken, whole grains, and low-fat dairy products. Additionally, don't forget to include healthy fats like nuts and olive oil, which can help reduce inflammation.

Organizing your shopping list is essential. Sort items into categories (produce, dairy, meats, and pantry staples) to make your trip to the store more productive. Before you go, check your pantry and refrigerator to make sure you have everything you need and to make sure you haven't bought anything twice. If you want to make the process even easier, consider using a shopping app or template.

When grocery shopping, it's important to be aware of potential triggers for gout and to steer clear of high-purine foods like red meat, organ meats, and shellfish, as well as sugary drinks and alcohol.

Following a gout-friendly diet can be made easier with effective meal prep. Begin by scheduling time each week to chop veggies, cook grains, and portion out proteins to expedite your cooking throughout the week. Use batch cooking to create large quantities of soups, stews, and casseroles that can be frozen or refrigerated for easy meals.

A well-organized kitchen can make it easier to stick to your meal plan and prevent you from reaching for unhealthy options when you're pressed for time. Use clear containers to store prepped ingredients and label them with the date to ensure freshness. Arrange your refrigerator and pantry to keep frequently used items easily accessible.

Meal prep can help you maintain a healthy, gout-friendly diet with less stress and effort throughout the week. Try new recipes and experiment with different cooking methods, such as grilling, roasting, and steaming.

OPTIONS FOR LOW-PURINE BREAKFAST

Low-purine breakfast foods are crucial for managing gout because they lower the body's uric acid levels. To kick off your day, make a cool fruit salad with low-purine fruits like cherries, apples, and berries. These fruits are rich in vitamins and antioxidants and can also help lower uric acid levels and inflammation. Serve your fruit salad with a slice of whole-grain toast that has been lightly topped with avocado for healthy fats and fiber.

Vegetable omelets made with egg substitutes are another great low-purine breakfast option. Use a variety of low-purine vegetables, like bell peppers, spinach, and tomatoes. Sauté the vegetables in a nonstick pan with a little olive oil, then add the egg substitute and cook until firm. This high-protein meal will satisfy you without adding more purines to your diet, which will help you effectively, manage your gout symptoms.

For a more conventional breakfast, consider a bowl of yogurt topped with chia seeds and low-purine fruits; to control purine levels, use nondairy yogurt substitutes like almond or coconut yogurt; this combination offers probiotics for gut health, fiber for digestion, and omega-3 fatty acids for inflammation reduction; it's an excellent way to start the day while following a gout-friendly diet.

JUICES AND SMOOTHIES FOR GOUT

Smoothies and juices are great choices for a quick and nourishing breakfast that helps manage gout. Start with a smoothie that contains frozen cherries, fresh kale, banana, and a small amount of almond milk; the cherries have anti-inflammatory and uric acid-lowering qualities, and the kale provides a healthy dose of vitamins and minerals.

Cucumbers and celery are great for a gout-friendly diet because they are low in purines and hydrating; lemon adds a zesty flavor and provides vitamin C, which can help lower uric acid levels.

Blend these ingredients and strain the juice to enjoy a light and energizing drink to start your day.

A different kind of smoothie is a berry and spinach blend. To make this, combine some strawberries, blueberries, and spinach with a dollop of Greek yogurt, a splash of water, or almond milk. The berries are high in vitamins and antioxidants, and the spinach adds necessary nutrients without supplying a lot of purines. This smoothie tastes great and also helps reduce inflammation and uric acid.

RECIPES FOR OATMEAL AND WHOLE GRAINS

For a gout-friendly breakfast, try these hearty and satisfying whole grain and oatmeal recipes: start with a bowl of steel-cut oats cooked in almond milk or water, then top with fresh fruits (like apples and blueberries) that are low in purines, and sprinkle with nuts (like walnuts or almonds) for extra protein and healthy fats.

Try a savory whole-grain breakfast bowl made with cooked quinoa in vegetable broth with sautéed spinach, cherry tomatoes, and avocado slices. Quinoa is a low-purine, complete protein, and a great option for a gout-friendly breakfast that is both filling and energizes you throughout the morning.

A buckwheat pancake is another delectable whole-grain recipe. Buckwheat is low in purines and gluten, so it's ideal for people with gout. To make the batter, combine buckwheat flour, water, baking powder, and cinnamon. Heat the mixture in a nonstick skillet until it's golden brown. Drizzle with pure maple syrup and fresh berries, and enjoy a satisfying breakfast that also helps keep your uric acid levels in check.

OTHER DAIRY AND EGG PRODUCTS

For those on a gout-friendly diet, egg and dairy substitutes are essential. Tofu scramble, for example, is a popular dish that mimics scrambled eggs without the high purine content. Toss firm tofu into a pan with sautéed onions, bell peppers, and spinach. Season with a pinch of salt, turmeric, and cumin for flavor.

This dish is full of protein and makes a delicious, gout-friendly breakfast.

Try almond or coconut yogurt, which is a dairy-free yogurt substitute that tastes creamy and is low in purines, making it a great option for gout management. Top with a handful of nuts, like almonds or walnuts, for crunch and nutrition, and low-purine fruits, like strawberries or peaches, to provide probiotics for gut health and essential nutrients to start your day off right.

Another great breakfast option is a chickpea omelet. To make the batter, mix the chickpea flour with water in a nonstick pan over medium heat. Add the sautéed vegetables (spinach, tomatoes, and mushrooms) and fold the omelet over; chickpea flour is low in purines and high in protein, so this is a great replacement for eggs for a gout-friendly breakfast.

IDEAS FOR A QUICK BREAKFAST

Avocado toast is a quick and nutritious breakfast option that is perfect for hectic mornings and can be easily modified to fit into a gout-friendly diet. Avocado is low in purines and provides healthy fats and fiber. Simply spread mashed avocado on a slice of whole-grain bread, top with sliced tomatoes, and sprinkle with salt and pepper.

Chia pudding is another quick and gout-friendly breakfast option. Simply combine chia seeds with almond milk and refrigerate overnight. Top the pudding with fresh berries and honey in the morning. Chia seeds are high in omega-3 fatty acids, which reduce inflammation, and low in purines. This prepped breakfast is not only convenient but also nutrient-dense, supporting a healthy start to your day.

A simple smoothie option is to blend a banana, a cup of almond milk, a handful of spinach, and a tablespoon of almond butter. This results in a high-nutrient, low-purine smoothie that is a great way for people with gout to get their recommended daily intake of protein, healthy fats, and carbohydrates.

GOUT-FRIENDLY RECIPES FOR SALADS

To make gout-friendly salads, start with a base of vitamin-rich, low-purine leafy greens like spinach, kale, or arugula. Add a variety of colorful vegetables, such as bell peppers, cucumbers, cherry tomatoes, and carrots, for extra nutrients and fiber. Finally, add fruits, like berries, apples, or pears, for a sweet contrast and extra antioxidants that are good for gout sufferers.

To keep purine levels in check, add lean protein sources to the salad (grilled chicken breast, turkey slices, or tofu are great options). If you're going plant-based, add a handful of chickpeas or black beans. To add crunch and healthy fats, sprinkle some nuts or seeds (almonds, sunflower seeds, or chia seeds are good options). If you dress your salad with a basic homemade vinaigrette (olive oil, lemon juice, and herbs), you can avoid the high-purine additives found in many store-bought dressings.

Try experimenting with different herbs and spices to add even more flavor to your salad. For example, fresh basil, cilantro, mint, or parsley can improve the flavor profile. To add texture, try adding avocado slices, boiled eggs, or a small amount of cheese, like goat cheese or feta.

These ingredients not only improve the flavor of your salad but also provide vital nutrients that support overall health and effectively manage symptoms of gout.

OPTIONS FOR LEAN PROTEIN

Lean protein choices are essential for gout management and overall health maintenance. Since poultry has less purine than red meat, it's a great choice. Choose skinless cuts and cook them using healthy techniques like grilling, baking, or steaming to reduce added fats. Fish, like salmon, is high in omega-3 fatty acids and low in purines, so it's a good option to include in moderation and provide anti-inflammatory benefits that can help manage gout.

Plant-based proteins are very helpful for people with gout. Legumes, like lentils, chickpeas, and black beans, are high in fiber and offer protein along with other nutrients that help with digestion and weight management. Tofu and tempeh are flexible protein options that work well in stir-fries and salads, as well as other recipes that call for meatless meat substitutes that fit in well with a gout-friendly diet.

Eggs are another fantastic source of low-purine protein; they can be included in a variety of recipes from breakfast to dinner, providing a versatile and nutritious addition to your gout diet. Dairy products can also be good sources of protein while being low in purines. Choose low-fat or fat-free options like Greek yogurt, cottage cheese, and milk. These can be used in breakfast dishes, snacks, or as part of main meals.

MAIN COURSES BASED ON VEGETABLES

One of the best ways to ensure that your diet is gout-friendly while still enjoying flavorful and satisfying meals is to make sure that your main dishes are made with vegetables. For example, a stuffed bell pepper filled with quinoa, black beans, corn, and tomatoes and seasoned with cumin and chili powder is a delicious and nutrient-dense meal. Start with hearty vegetables like eggplant, zucchini, and mushrooms.

Add a base of tofu or tempeh for protein and stir-fry in a small amount of olive oil with garlic, ginger, and soy sauce for flavor. Serve over brown rice or whole grain noodles to keep the dish balanced and filling. The combination of textures and flavors will not only be satisfying but will also adhere to a low-purine diet. Stir-fries are another great option that combines a variety of vegetables like broccoli, bell peppers, snap peas, and carrots.

Another fantastic and simple main dish is a vegetable casserole. Layers of thinly sliced potatoes, zucchini, and tomatoes are combined, and then cheese and fresh herbs are sprinkled on top. Bake until the vegetables are soft and the cheese is golden. This dish can be made ahead of time and reheated, which makes it a great weeknight meal. Vegetable-based dishes are so versatile that you can make as many variations as you want to keep your gout diet interesting and varied.

RECIPES FOR LOW-PURINE SOUPS & STEWS

Rich in vitamins and minerals but low in purines, soups, and stews can be a nourishing and comforting part of a gout-friendly diet. Begin with a base of vegetables, such as onions, carrots, celery, and garlic, sautéed in olive oil; add low-purine broth, such as vegetable or chicken broth, to create a flavorful foundation; add a variety of vegetables, such as tomatoes, bell peppers, zucchini, and leafy greens.

Add legumes (lentils, chickpeas, or black beans) for protein; these are low in purines and provide heartiness and nutrition; you can also add tofu for an additional plant-based protein source; season the soup or stew with herbs and spices (paprika, cumin, thyme, rosemary) to bring out the flavor without adding extra high-purine ingredients; a squeeze of lemon juice or vinegar brightens the meal.

This is a great way to make gout-friendly stews because it slowly cooks the flavors and keeps the vegetables and legumes tender. To make a vegetable and barley stew, add diced tomatoes, carrots, celery, and barley to vegetable broth along with your preferred seasonings. Simmer until the ingredients are soft and the flavors are well combined. This filling stew can be made in big batches and frozen for easy, nutritious meals all week long.

TECHNIQUES FOR GRILLING AND ROASTING

The healthy cooking techniques of grilling and roasting can bring out the flavor of gout-friendly foods without adding too much fat.

For grilling, opt for lean meats like turkey, chicken breasts, or fish, and marinate the proteins in a marinade of olive oil, lemon juice, garlic, and herbs to add flavor without raising the levels of purines. Use an outdoor grill pan or grill pan, and make sure the meat is cooked through but not burned, as this can increase the amount of harmful compounds.

Slicing bell peppers, zucchini, eggplant, and asparagus, tossing them in olive oil with a pinch of salt, pepper, and your preferred herbs, and grilling them until they are soft and have nice grill marks, or roasting them by spreading the seasoned vegetables on a baking sheet and baking at a high temperature until they are caramelized and slightly crispy, are other ways that vegetables lend themselves to grilling and roasting.

A great way to incorporate lean proteins and veggies into your meals is to make mixed skewers: alternately, put pieces of chicken or tofu with chunks of onion, bell pepper, cherry tomatoes, and mushrooms. Brush the skewers with a light marinade and grill until the ingredients are cooked through. This method looks good and guarantees a balanced intake of proteins and vegetables, which will help you follow a gout-friendly diet while still enjoying tasty, nourishing meals.

HEALTHY SNACK SUGGESTIONS

Nuts and seeds, like walnuts and flaxseeds, provide healthy fats and can be sprinkled over salads or eaten on their own. Vegetables, like celery, carrots, and bell peppers, make excellent snacks when paired with hummus or a light dressing.

Start with fruits, like cherries, strawberries, and blueberries, which are known for their anti-inflammatory qualities and can be enjoyed fresh or blended into smoothies with low-fat yogurt or almond milk.

A great snack combination is whole grain crackers with cottage cheese or low-fat cheese; whole grains also help to stabilize blood sugar, which is advantageous for people with gout; hard-boiled eggs are a portable, high-protein snack; adding legumes, such as edamame, can also provide an additional source of protein without the purine content of animal products.

Finally, for a filling and healthy snack, try creating a batch of homemade granola bars with oats, honey, and dried fruits. Instead of using high-purine ingredients like peanuts or sunflower seeds, try using almonds or pumpkin seeds. These snacks are healthy and convenient because they can be made ahead of time and kept in the fridge for easy access all week.

SPREADS AND DIPS SAFE FOR GOUT

When making dips and spreads, it's important to use ingredients that are high in nutrients and low in purines. A classic hummus made with chickpeas, tahini, lemon juice, and garlic is a great example of this. The combination of flavors in the hummus makes it a satisfying and nourishing dip, and fresh veggies like cucumber slices, cherry tomatoes, and bell peppers pair well with it.

Avocado-based guacamole is another spread that's good for gout sufferers. Rich in healthy fats and low in purines, avocados can help reduce inflammation. To make basic guacamole, mash ripe avocados with diced tomatoes, chopped cilantro, lime juice, and a dash of salt. This spread is versatile enough to go well with fish or chicken on the grill or with whole-grain crackers.

Try a yogurt and fruit dip instead; just combine low-fat Greek yogurt with a little honey and a few fresh berries or sliced peaches. This dip is a great way to satisfy your sweet tooth while also consuming probiotics and antioxidants that are good for your general health. These gout-safe spreads and dips are simple to include in your regular meals and offer tasty and healthy options.

SNACKS FOR PARTIES AND FINGER FOODS

It can be difficult to host a party or get-together while following a gout-friendly diet, but there are lots of delicious finger foods and snacks that will appeal to all tastes. Start with vegetable skewers, which are colorful, refreshing, and low in purines. They are made from cherry tomatoes, cucumber slices, and bell pepper chunks and are drizzled with olive oil and sprinkled with herbs.

An even better option would be turkey or chicken meatballs, which are made with lean ground meat and combined with egg, breadcrumbs, minced garlic, and your preferred herbs. These meatballs are healthy enough to bake rather than fry, and they go well with a homemade tomato sauce made with fresh tomatoes, garlic, and basil for dipping. These meatballs are gout-friendly and delicious, so they'll be a hit at any gathering.

To add some sweetness, make fruit kebabs with a range of fresh fruits, including grapes, pineapple, strawberries, and melon. Using skewers, arrange the fruit pieces to create a visually appealing and easy-to-eat snack. Serve these with a light yogurt dip flavored with a hint of honey and vanilla extract. These finger foods and party snacks are not only delicious but also fit for guests with gout.

EASY APPETIZERS FOR EVERY EVENT

A simple yet elegant appetizer that is both gout-friendly and pleasing to large groups of people is smoked salmon on whole grain toast points. Toss a slice of smoked salmon, top with a dollop of low-fat cream cheese, and garnish with fresh dill. This appetizer comes together quickly and offers a healthy balance of fats and protein without being overly purine-filled.

Another delicious and easy appetizer is stuffed mushrooms. Start with large button mushrooms, trim the stems, and stuff the caps with a filling of low-fat cream cheese, chopped spinach, garlic, and a little Parmesan cheese. Bake until the filling is golden brown and the mushrooms are soft. These stuffed mushrooms are a hit for any kind of gathering.

Serve cucumber bites with a light tuna salad for a cool alternative. Combine canned tuna, a tiny bit of low-fat mayonnaise, chopped celery, and a squeeze of lemon juice. Cut cucumbers into thick rounds and place a spoonful of the tuna mixture on top of each slice. Add some fresh dill or chives for flavor. These simple appetizers go well with a gout-friendly diet and are a hit at any gathering.

It can be satisfying and fun to find gout-friendly dessert substitutes. Baked apples, which are naturally sweet and offer a comforting treat without the high purine content of many traditional desserts, are one such option. Core the apples and fill them with a mixture of oats, honey, and cinnamon. Bake until soft and serve warm.

Chia seed pudding is another fantastic dessert option. To make it, mix chia seeds with almond milk and a small amount of vanilla extract. Cover and refrigerate overnight until the mixture becomes pudding-like. Garnish with honey or fresh berries for extra sweetness. Rich in fiber and omega-3 fatty acids, chia seed pudding is a gout-friendly and healthy dessert choice.

Finally, try creating a fruit sorbet with seasonal, fresh fruit. Simply blend mangoes, strawberries, or peaches with a little lemon juice and honey, freeze until solid, then blend again until smooth.

TIPS FOR HYDRATION IN GOUT MANAGEMENT

Drinking plenty of water is essential for managing gout. It flushes out uric acid from the body, which lowers the chance of crystal formation in the joints. Try to drink eight glasses or more of water per day, but if you live in a hot climate or engage in strenuous activity, you should drink more.

You can also include foods high in water, like cucumbers, watermelons, and strawberries, in your diet to further increase your water intake.

To make sure you're meeting your hydration goals, it's also a good idea to track how much fluid you consume throughout the day. You can do this by setting reminders on your phone or using a water-tracking app. Sugary drinks and sodas should be avoided as they can raise uric acid levels and aggravate gout symptoms. Instead, go for natural options like coconut water, which is not only hydrating but also contains electrolytes that can help maintain a healthy balance in your body.

Slices of fruit (lemon, lime, berries) can add natural flavor to your water to make it more appealing and help you meet your hydration goals.

Herbal teas are another good addition because they are a good source of hydration without adding calories or sugar, which makes them a good choice for managing gout.

GOUT-FRIENDLY SHAKES & SMOOTHIES

Blending a base of low-fat or non-dairy milk, like almond milk or coconut milk, which are less likely to trigger gout symptoms compared to high-fat dairy products, with leafy greens like spinach or kale, which are rich in antioxidants and can help reduce inflammation, is a delicious way to manage your condition while enjoying a variety of nutrients.

Add fruits with lower fructose content, like berries, which are also high in vitamin C and other nutrients;

stay away from high fructose fruits, like apples and pears, as they can raise uric acid levels; and for extra taste and nutrition, add seeds, like flaxseeds or chia, which are high in fiber and omega-3 fatty acids that can help with overall health and reduce inflammation.

For optimal flavor and nutritional value, blend until smooth and consume right away. These smoothies can be a healthy breakfast option or a light snack that complements your gout treatment regimen. Try blending different combinations of fruits and greens to create recipes that you enjoy and that is good for your gout.

HERBAL INFUSIONS AND TEAS

Herbal teas and infusions can be a calming and useful way to manage the symptoms of gout. Some herbs are good to include in a gout diet because they have uric acid-lowering and anti-inflammatory properties.

For example, nettle tea has been used traditionally to reduce joint pain and inflammation; make a cup by steeping dried nettle leaves in hot water for about 10 minutes.

Turmeric tea, which is made by simmering turmeric powder or fresh turmeric root in water, is also highly recommended for its anti-inflammatory effects and ability to lower uric acid levels.

Another beneficial herbal tea is ginger tea, which is known for its potent anti-inflammatory properties. To make it, simply slice fresh ginger root and steep it in boiling water for 10-15 minutes. You can also add a little honey or lemon to enhance the flavor.

These herbal teas, which support hydration and offer a range of health benefits, can help manage gout symptoms and offer a soothing beverage option when included in your daily routine. You can drink them hot or iced, depending on your preference, and try different herbs to see which ones work best for you.

To effectively manage gout, it is imperative to comprehend the relationship between alcohol and gout. Specifically, drinking beer and spirits can raise blood levels of uric acid, which can exacerbate gout symptoms. Beer contains purines, which the body converts to uric acid. Conversely, drinking spirits can impair the kidneys' capacity to eliminate uric acid, which can raise blood levels of the mineral even further.

If you do choose to drink, moderation is key. Have one or two drinks on special occasions, and always choose low-purine options (wine, for example, has less of an effect on uric acid levels than beer). If you are experiencing a flare-up of gout, stay away from alcohol completely to avoid exacerbating your symptoms.

You can better manage your gout and lessen the frequency and severity of flare-ups by choosing mindfully what alcohol to drink. Some satisfying healthy substitutes for alcoholic beverages are herbal iced teas, sparkling water with a splash of fruit juice, and non-alcoholic cocktails made with fresh ingredients.

RECIPES FOR HYDRATION

A refreshing cucumber and mint water is a great place to start when creating hydration recipes for gout management. Simply slice half a cucumber and add a handful of fresh mint leaves to a pitcher of water, cover, and refrigerate for a few hours before drinking. This combination tastes great and offers extra hydration and a cooling effect.

Try a berry-infused water for a more nutrient-dense option. In a large jug of water, combine a mixture of strawberries, blueberries, and raspberries with a few slices of lemon. Let the flavors meld in the refrigerator for a few hours. The antioxidant-rich berries not only add a touch of sweetness but also support overall health by reducing inflammation.

These easy yet effective recipes can make staying hydrated enjoyable and beneficial for your gout management plan. Another great hydration recipe is coconut water with a twist of lime. Just pour fresh coconut water into a glass and squeeze in the juice of one lime. This drink is not only hydrating but also replenishes electrolytes, making it an ideal choice for gout sufferers, especially after exercise or on a hot day.

CHAPTER FOUR

GOUT-FRIENDLY CHRISTMAS DINNERS

It can be a happy and fulfilling experience to prepare gout-friendly holiday meals, which let you enjoy the flavors of the season without risking a flare-up. Start with low-purine appetizers, like stuffed mushrooms or roasted vegetable platters; lean proteins, like baked salmon or roasted turkey, seasoned with herbs and spices rather than rich sauces; and for sides, try delicious and nutritious quinoa salad with cranberries and nuts or sweet potato mash.

If you're thinking about desserts, go for low-sugar and low-purine options. Lime-dressed fresh fruit salads or cinnamon-topped baked apples make great meal finales. Make sure your dishes have lots of vibrant vegetables and whole grains for a well-rounded and filling spread. When cooking, use olive oil rather than butter—it's a healthier fat choice.

Prepare a gout-friendly meal without sacrificing flavor or festiveness. Careful planning and inventive preparation can result in a holiday feast that is safe for your condition and delicious. To make your meals even more memorable, set a beautiful table with festive decorations and concentrate on the company of your loved ones.

IDEAS FOR A CELEBRATORY DINNER

When planning a menu for celebratory dinners, it's important to create an indulgent yet safe dish for gout sufferers. Start with a light soup, like a chilled cucumber and dill soup, or a light vegetable consommé, and work your way up to a main course like grilled chicken breast served with roasted asparagus and barley risotto. These dishes are elegant, high in nutrients, and low in purines—perfect for a special occasion.

To keep the meal interesting, add a variety of flavors and textures. For example, a side salad of mixed greens, avocado, and lemon vinaigrette can bring brightness and freshness. For dessert, try something different, like poached pears in red wine (the alcohol is cooked off) or a dairy-free sorbet made with fresh berries and mint; these are sophisticated and suitable for people with gout.

Just as important as the food is creating a welcoming atmosphere; light candles, use your finest dinnerware, play soothing background music, and make the dining experience truly memorable. By emphasizing quality ingredients and careful preparation, you can create a celebratory dinner that is both dietary-conscious and unforgettable.

OPTIONS FOR A PICNIC AND POTLUCK

With the right recipes, organizing a gout-friendly picnic or potluck can be stress-free and enjoyable. Start with finger food, such as hummus with vegetable sticks or whole-grain crackers topped with avocado and cherry tomatoes; these portable appetizers are tasty and nutritious.

For the main course, try a quinoa and vegetable salad or a chickpea and spinach wrap; these dishes are simple to make, transport, and share.

Drinks: Steer clear of alcohol and sugar-filled sodas; instead, try refreshing drinks like iced herbal teas or cucumber-mint-infused water. If you're in the mood for something sweet, pack some fresh fruit skewers or make some homemade granola bars with oats, almonds, and dried fruits. They're satisfying and won't make your gout flare-up worse.

With these gout-friendly options, you can have a fun picnic or potluck without worrying about your diet. Don't forget to pack plenty of utensils, napkins, and a cooler to keep everything fresh. You can also make a cozy picnic area with blankets and cushions.

MENUS FOR BIRTHDAYS AND ANNIVERSARIES

Birthdays and anniversaries require a menu that is both celebratory and sensitive to dietary needs. Begin with sophisticated appetizers like a caprese salad with fresh mozzarella, tomatoes, and basil or a shrimp cocktail with a light lemon dressing. For the main course, try baked salmon with a dill and lemon sauce, served with roasted Brussels sprouts and wild rice pilaf. Both of these dishes are sophisticated and low in purines, making them ideal for a celebratory meal.

For dessert, try something different like a flourless almond cake or a berry parfait with Greek yogurt and honey. Both of these desserts are great for people with gout. To keep the celebration light and fun, pair your meal with sparkling water infused with citrus slices or a glass of non-alcoholic wine.

Adorn your dining space with flowers and sentimental touches that correspond with the significance of the occasion.

FESTIVE AND SEASONAL RECIPES

Festive and seasonal recipes can be made gout-friendly without sacrificing their appeal. For example, in springtime, try a light asparagus and pea risotto or a grilled chicken with lemon and herbs. In summer, try fresh salads made with ingredients like watermelon, feta, and mint, or grilled vegetable kebabs. These recipes highlight seasonal produce while keeping purine levels in check.

Fall menus can include hearty dishes like roasted root vegetables with quinoa or butternut squash soup as the weather cools. For winter celebrations, consider slow-cooked dishes like a vegetable stew or a baked apple dessert with walnuts and cinnamon. These warm, comforting dishes are ideal for enjoying the season without aggravating your gout.

Make your meal feel special by using themed centerpieces, vibrant napkins, and seasonal flowers. These gout-friendly seasonal recipes allow you to enjoy the flavors and customs of each season without sacrificing your health. Incorporate seasonal decorations and table settings to heighten the festive atmosphere.

CHAPTER FIVE

HANDLING FLARES OF GOUT

HOW TO IDENTIFY GOUT SYMPTOMS

Understanding these symptoms helps you distinguish a gout attack from other types of joint pain and enables timely intervention. Gout typically presents with sudden and severe pain in a joint, usually the big toe. This pain can be so intense that it wakes you up. It may also be accompanied by swelling, redness, and warmth in the affected area. The skin around the joint can also appear shiny and peel as the flare progresses.

Other than the big toe, gout can also affect the ankles, knees, elbows, wrists, and fingers. It usually flares up quickly, peaking in less than a day. When the joint flares up, it can become so tender that even the weight of a bed sheet can cause excruciating pain. If you recognize these symptoms, you can seek medical attention as soon as possible and start treatment, which will lessen the length and intensity of the attack.

Understanding the early signs and symptoms of gout is the first step in managing this condition and preventing future flare-ups. In some cases, gout symptoms can be accompanied by fever and malaise, which can be mistaken for an infection. Monitoring your symptoms and keeping a record of their frequency, duration, and triggers can help your healthcare provider diagnose gout accurately and tailor your treatment plan effectively.

QUICK DIETARY CHANGES

During a flare-up, dietary changes should be made as soon as possible to reduce symptoms and stop future attacks. Foods high in purines should be avoided as they raise uric acid levels and aggravate symptoms of gout. Red meats, organ meats, shellfish, and some fish, such as sardines and mackerel, should be reduced or avoided. Low-purine foods, such as legumes, tofu, and low-fat dairy products, can help control uric acid levels.

Apart from limiting your intake of high-purine foods, it's also important to include foods that are known to be anti-inflammatory.

Fresh fruits, especially cherries, strawberries, and blueberries, have been shown to have anti-inflammatory qualities and may help lessen the intensity of gout symptoms. Whole grains, nuts, and vegetables are also important additions to your meals as they offer vital nutrients and promote general health. These simple dietary adjustments can have a big impact on controlling a flare-up and speeding up the healing process.

Drinking plenty of water can help flush out excess uric acid from the body, reducing the risk of crystal formation in the joints. You can also get your fluid intake from herbal teas and diluted fruit juices, which don't add extra calories or sugar. By making these dietary adjustments as soon as possible, you can effectively manage gout flare-ups and minimize their impact on your daily life.

THINGS NOT TO EAT WHILE FLARING

It is important to avoid certain foods during a flare-up to avoid making the condition worse. The main culprits are high-purine foods, which raise blood uric acid levels. Red meats, like beef, pork, and lamb, as well as organ meats, like liver and kidneys, should be strictly avoided. Seafood, like shrimp, lobster, and anchovies, can also cause flare-ups, so avoid them.

In addition, alcohol—especially beer and spirits—can aggravate the symptoms of gout by interfering with the body's ability to excrete uric acid, which can result in elevated levels and the formation of crystals in the joints.

To prevent aggravating symptoms, avoid alcohol completely during a gout flare-up; instead, drink plenty of water, herbal teas, and other non-alcoholic beverages to stay hydrated and promote uric acid excretion.

Processed foods and refined carbohydrates, such as white bread, pasta, and pastries, should also be avoided. By doing so, you can help manage gout flares more effectively and reduce the severity and duration of symptoms. Sugary foods and beverages, including sodas, fruit juices, and desserts, should also be limited during a gout flare. These items can increase uric acid production and contribute to inflammation.

TIPS FOR HYDRATION AND REST

Maintaining adequate hydration levels is important for managing flare-ups of gout because water dilutes uric acid and prevents crystal formation in the joints. Herbal teas and broth-based soups can also help you stay hydrated. Sugary and caffeinated beverages should be avoided as they can dehydrate you and aggravate gout symptoms. Eight glasses of water a day is the recommended minimum amount of water to drink.

Elevating the affected limb can help reduce swelling and improve comfort. Using supportive devices like a brace or splint can provide additional stability to the joint, minimizing movement and pain. Applying ice packs for 15-20 minutes several times a day can also help reduce inflammation and numb the area, providing relief from severe pain. Rest is equally important during a gout flare.

Once the acute pain has subsided, gentle exercises and stretches may be helpful. Low-impact activities such as swimming or cycling can enhance joint flexibility and general health without placing undue strain on the affected joint.

The key to effectively managing flare-ups and averting more attacks is to maintain a balance between rest and activity. You can also support your body's healing process and effectively manage gout symptoms by staying hydrated and allowing ample rest.

PLAN FOR RECUPERATION DIET

After a flare-up, you should create a recovery diet plan to avoid more flare-ups and to keep your health in check. You should emphasize eating foods high in nutrients and low in purines; you should also make fresh fruits and vegetables—especially those that have anti-inflammatory qualities like cherries and leafy greens—a mainstay of your diet; and whole grains, like oats, brown rice, and quinoa, offer important nutrients and fiber without raising your uric acid levels.

Healthy fats from sources like avocados, nuts, and olive oil can also support overall health and reduce inflammation. Lean proteins are a key component of a recovery diet. Choose plant-based proteins like beans, lentils, and tofu, as well as low-fat dairy products. These options provide the necessary protein without the high purine content found in red and organ meats.

Long-term strategies for your recovery diet include drinking plenty of water, avoiding alcohol and sugar-filled drinks, and drinking herbal teas, and eating foods high in water, like watermelon and cucumbers. You can also significantly lower your chance of future gout flare-ups by regularly checking your uric acid levels and eating a balanced diet, which will help you manage your condition more effectively and live a better quality of life.

CHAPTER SIX

LIFESTYLE SUGGESTIONS TO PREVENT GOUT

EXERCISE AND GUIDELINES FOR PHYSICAL ACTIVITY

Engaging in low-impact activities like walking, swimming, or cycling can be especially helpful as they minimize joint stress while promoting cardiovascular health. Aim for at least 150 minutes of moderate aerobic activity per week, broken into manageable sessions. Strength training exercises, performed twice or three times a week, can also enhance muscle mass and joint stability, further supporting overall health. Regular exercise is essential in preventing gout flare-ups by helping maintain a healthy weight and reducing uric acid levels.

Flexibility and balance exercises, such as yoga or tai chi, can enhance joint function and lower the risk of falls or injuries. These activities not only improve physical health but also lower stress levels, which benefits mental health.

If you're new to exercising, begin slowly and build up to longer and more intense workouts to prevent overdoing it. A certified fitness trainer or healthcare professional can help customize an exercise program that meets your needs and abilities.

Staying hydrated, dressing appropriately, warming up and cooling down after workouts can help prevent injuries and ensure a safe, effective workout routine. Remember, consistency is key to reaping the long-term benefits of regular physical activity. It's important to listen to your body and avoid activities that cause pain or discomfort, especially during a gout attack.

TECHNIQUES FOR STRESS MANAGEMENT

Effective stress management is essential for preventing gout because stress can aggravate symptoms and cause inflammation. Deep breathing exercises, meditation, and progressive muscle relaxation are a few relaxation techniques that can help reduce stress and calm the mind.

These techniques are simple to incorporate into daily routines and offer both short-term relief and long-term mental health benefits.

Stress management can also be greatly aided by hobbies and fulfilling pursuits. Whether it's reading, painting, gardening, or learning to play an instrument, spending time on enjoyable activities can divert attention from everyday concerns and lift one's spirits. Social relationships are also crucial; having close bonds with friends and family offers emotional support and reduces the negative effects of stress.

Setting realistic goals, prioritizing tasks, and scheduling downtime for self-care and relaxation can all help prevent feelings of overwhelm. Seeking professional assistance from a therapist or counselor can also help reduce chronic stress and ultimately improve gout management. Lastly, creating a structured daily routine can help reduce stress by giving one a sense of control and predictability.

Achieving seven to nine hours of quality sleep every night by creating a regular sleep schedule is important for managing gout because it allows the body to repair and reduces inflammation. Getting to bed and waking up at the same time every day, including on weekends, can help regulate the body's internal clock and improve the quality of sleep. Creating a comfortable and distraction-free sleep environment also helps promote better sleep.

Developing a relaxing pre-sleep routine, like reading, taking a warm bath, or gently stretching, can signal to the body that it's time to wind down. Limiting exposure to screens and electronic devices before bed can also help, as the blue light emitted can interfere with the production of melatonin, the sleep hormone. Ultimately, achieving restorative rest depends on practicing good sleep hygiene.

Prioritizing sleep not only supports overall health but also plays a crucial role in preventing flare-ups and effectively managing symptoms. For those who are having trouble sleeping due to pain or discomfort from gout, using supportive pillows and maintaining a comfortable sleeping position can help. Consulting with a healthcare provider about potential sleep aids or pain management strategies might be necessary.

VITAMINS & SUPPLEMENTS FOR GOUT

Vitamin C, for example, has been shown to lower blood levels of uric acid, making it a useful addition to a gout-preventive diet. Aim to include more vitamin C-rich foods such as oranges, strawberries, and bell peppers, or consider taking a daily supplement as directed by a healthcare provider. Certain vitamins and supplements can help prevent and manage gout by reducing uric acid levels and inflammation.

Additionally, cherries and cherry extract supplements have been linked to lower uric acid levels and fewer flare-ups with gout, making them a useful dietary addition. Omega-3 fatty acids, found in fish oil supplements, have anti-inflammatory properties that can help reduce the frequency and severity of gout attacks. You can get these beneficial nutrients by eating fatty fish like salmon and mackerel or by taking a high-quality fish oil supplement.

A well-rounded approach to managing and preventing gout can be achieved by combining the right supplements with a balanced diet high in fruits, vegetables, whole grains, and lean proteins. Never start taking new supplements without first consulting a healthcare provider, as they may interact with medications or have contraindications based on specific health conditions.

MONITORING DEVELOPMENT AND MODIFICATIONS

Monitoring dietary intake, exercise routines, stress levels, sleep patterns, and any flare-ups of gout can help you identify patterns and make necessary adjustments to your treatment plan. Furthermore, keeping a thorough journal can help you gain valuable insights into what triggers symptoms and what strategies work best for managing them.

Having regular check-ups with healthcare providers is essential for assessing the patient's progress and making well-informed decisions regarding treatment modifications. Objective data to inform management strategies can be obtained through joint health assessments and blood tests to monitor uric acid levels; based on these results, medical professionals can recommend dietary, exercise, or medication regimen modifications to optimize gout control.

Long-term success in managing gout requires flexibility and adaptability. As lifestyle habits change and new challenges emerge, it's important to be open to modifying strategies to ensure continued progress and symptom control. People with gout can effectively manage their condition and improve their overall quality of life by remaining proactive, informed, and involved in self-care practices.

CHAPTER SEVEN

CAN SOMEONE WITH GOUT EAT SEAFOOD?

The problem with seafood for gout sufferers is that a lot of it has high purine content, which the body converts to uric acid. Since uric acid can trigger gout attacks, it's important to choose your seafood carefully.

Shrimp, lobster, and some fish, like anchovies and sardines, have a lot of purines and should be eaten in moderation; salmon, tilapia, and trout, on the other hand, have fewer purines and should be consumed occasionally.

If you're going to cook seafood, try grilling, baking, or steaming it instead of frying it. This will keep the dish healthier and less likely to cause gout symptoms. You can balance your meal and cut down on purines by serving seafood with lots of vegetables. Eating fish that's high in omega-3s, like salmon, in moderation can also help reduce inflammation and manage gout symptoms.

Not only is it important to watch portion sizes, but you can also enjoy seafood without significantly increasing your risk of a flare-up by including small portions of low-purine seafood into a well-balanced diet rather than consuming large amounts at once.

HOW FREQUENTLY SHOULD I CHECK MY LEVELS OF URIC ACID?

Effective gout management requires regular monitoring of your uric acid levels. Your doctor may initially advise testing every few months to establish a baseline and assess how well your treatment plan is working. Once your uric acid levels are stable and within the target range, you may only need to test once or twice a year; however, more frequent testing may be required if you have a history of gout attacks or if your symptoms have changed.

A basic blood test is usually used to measure the amount of uric acid in your blood and determine your risk of developing gout or experiencing a flare-up of gout.

It is recommended to have the test done following a fast because some foods and drinks have the potential to temporarily raise uric acid levels. You should talk to your healthcare provider about the best times to schedule these tests to get accurate results.

Apart from routine testing, it can be helpful to maintain a symptom diary where you record any dietary modifications, medication use, and flare-ups. This will help your doctor decide on the best course of action for your treatment and may identify certain triggers that you should stay away from to better control your gout.

DOES COFFEE HELP WITH GOUT?

Studies have indicated that regular coffee consumption may lower the risk of developing gout by reducing uric acid levels; this effect is thought to be due to the antioxidant properties of coffee and its ability to improve insulin sensitivity, which helps lower uric acid production. Coffee has been a topic of interest about gout, and research suggests that it might have a beneficial effect.

Drinking up to three to four cups of coffee a day is generally regarded as safe and may even help reduce the frequency of gout attacks for those who are already managing their gout. However, it's important to avoid adding excessive sugar or high-fat creamers to your coffee, as these can counteract the benefits and contribute to weight gain, which is a risk factor for gout. Moderate coffee consumption can be part of a healthy diet.

Coffee has potential health benefits, but it's also important to stay hydrated. Drink plenty of water throughout the day to avoid dehydration, which can raise uric acid levels and cause gout attacks. You can enjoy the benefits of coffee without aggravating gout symptoms by balancing your intake of coffee and water.

WHICH SNACKS ARE IDEAL FOR GOUT?

To effectively manage gout, it's important to choose snacks that are rich in nutrients that help reduce inflammation and low in purines. Fresh fruits, such as berries, apples, and cherries, are great options because of their anti-inflammatory qualities, which have been shown to lower uric acid levels and reduce the risk of gout attacks.

When paired with a healthy dip like hummus, vegetables like carrot sticks, cucumber slices, and bell pepper strips make satisfying low-purine snacks that are also high in vitamins and minerals. Nuts and seeds like flaxseeds, walnuts, and almonds also work well as low-purine snacks because they are high in healthy fats that can help reduce inflammation.

If you'd like something more substantial, whole-grain crackers with a dab of peanut butter or avocado can be a satisfying and nutritious snack.

By selecting these kinds of snacks, you can effectively manage your gout while still indulging in delicious and satisfying treats. Low-fat dairy products, such as yogurt or cheese, can help lower uric acid levels and provide calcium and vitamin D.

Dealing with social situations when you have gout can be difficult, but it can be managed with some preparation and communication. If you attend events or eat out, let your host or server know that you have gout-related dietary restrictions. This will help to ensure that appropriate food options are available and that most people will be understanding and accommodating.

Take into account eating a small, gout-friendly meal before you go to help stave off temptation from high-purine foods. Another tactic is to bring a dish to share that you know is safe for you to eat, which not only assures you of having something to eat but also introduces others to delectable, gout-friendly cuisine.

Alcohol consumption should be limited because it raises uric acid levels. Instead, choose water, herbal teas, or non-alcoholic beverages, and stay hydrated during the event.

www.ingramcontent.com/pod-product-compliance
Lightning Source LLC
Chambersburg PA
CBHW050652250726
48662CB00002B/626